$9.95

Fountain Of Youth Formula™ Overview Report

New!

Miracle Cure!

Natural Cures

Truly amazing!
Works in minutes!
Guaranteed!

BANNED IN THE USA

Fountain Of Youth Formula™:
Overview Report

Ron Benson

Published by Ron Benson, Creative Director, Paladin Movies International 2016.

FOUNTAIN OF YOUTH FORMULA™: OVERVIEW REPORT

First edition. January 24, 2016.

ISBN-13: 978-1523727605

ISBN-10: 1523727608

Written by Ron Benson.

TABLE OF CONTENTS

I *INTRODUCTION*

Do you know it has been scientifically proven that you can cure virtually all diseases with natural therapies and also stop the aging process? Are you interested in knowing how to stop growing old and learning how to grow young instead?

If so you are very fortunate, because I don't live in the USA anymore where most natural cures and therapies are banned. So I no longer have to worry about being Blacklisted... Exiled... Bankrupted... Criminalized... or ending up in Jail, and I am free to tell you the whole truth and nothing but the truth!

The inspiration to publish the *Fountain Of Youth Formula*™ is due to the unnecessary loss of family, friends, and loved one's because of the lies and deception, and especially the ban on safe and proven natural cures in the USA. Much of the *Fountain Of Youth Formula*™ is based on my life long personal experiences, but mostly due to being Blessed to be a World Trade Center disaster survivor who has physically recovered. Strange as it may sound I was Blessed to get injured on the job and crippled when working at the World Trade Center, so I was off work the day the buildings came down.

That is called Blessing Through Adversity, because I have been able to fully recover physically from being crippled unable to use my left arm or walk without a crutch. My left arm was finished and required arthroscopic surgery, but I was able to avoid surgery on my back and right knee. After I was crippled I lost both of my jobs then I became homeless in NYC, so I thought that I was a cursed man. But on the day of the disaster even though my left arm was useless in a sling and I was using a crutch for my right leg I struggled to get past the hordes of gray soot covered people who looked like zombies as they were escaping from the Twin Towers on the Brooklyn Bridge.

I was trying to get to the Twin Towers and help with the rescue efforts, because among many other good people and associates I also lost a woman who I loved and one of my best friends who I had gotten hired on the job that day. It was then that I realized I was Blessed to get crippled on the job and to be alive. So I stopped feeling sorry for myself, prayed for those who were lost, and joined the relief crew to assist those who had escaped the disaster. I also became convicted to doing the best I could to rehab my body, even though I became homeless. Fortunately in the past I was a Physical Education instructor at Chicago State University, and with the help of the great Physical Therapists at Bellevue Hospital in NYC I started working on my physical recovery. Although progress was slow, since I also had severe depression and anxiety.

After more than a year of encouragement "Saint" Vincent Wallace who is one of my best life long friends and a Kappa Alpha Psi Fraternity Brother finally convinced me to come back to Los Angeles, where I was able to fully recover physically and get a new life. The journey to full physical recovery was a full time job that took 5+ years. It required 2 days of physical therapy provided by the great Physical Therapists at the King/Drew Hospital in Los Angeles, and 3 to 4 days of working out every week, plus mega vitamin and juicing therapies. BTW I was also injured and crippled again in 2015, but I was able to avoid surgery again. So I am still a living testimony of Blessing Through Adversity and for the power and effectiveness of natural therapies.

You don't have to take my word for anything because there is documented publicly available proof for the *Fountain Of Youth Formula*™, that is easily accessible for almost everyone who has a cellphone these days. So this life saving and enhancing information can not be suppressed and censored any longer, as it has been for many decades in the past.

The first video in the next section made me extremely angry because the FDA is locking people up in jail who are promoting natural cures, as if the FDA really cares about protecting the people's health. If the FDA really cared about protecting people's health the FDA would have locked up some of the medical scam artists who have been over diagnosing and charging people $100 billion per year for unnecessary and toxic chemotherapy treatments:
http://www.naturalnews.com/051482_cancer_industry_overdiagnosis_false_positi
ves.html

A few of the videos in the next section made me so angry they brought tears to my eyes and almost made me cry even though I am still a soldier who has been trained to be stoic no matter if I am bleeding or being beaten. But it is so sad to see that the health care industry in the USA cares more about profits, than for the health of our children, family, and friends. It is as if they think they can take the money with them to Hell and spend it.

Fortunately there is lots of good news and even though *The Technological Revolution Is Not Being Televised*™: http://blog.paladinmovies.com/2015/12/newviralsocialtech masses of people are still being empowered globally. Never before now did the average person have access to communication, information, creative capabilities, and business opportunities, that are now available and easily accessible for anyone with a modern cellphone. As a result this is the prime time to utilize the *Fountain Of Youth Formula*™ to be healthy, live long, prosper, and most importantly to do good works and Be Blessed!

Even so due to the current state of the world you may be pessimistic about prospects for the future. So the last 2 videos by Dr. Julian Simon and Paladin Movies International are provided to give you hope and inspiration about the future, because there are solutions to Change The World For The Better! Dr. Julian Simon proved population is the ultimate resource, and that the so-called theories about over population and the scarcity of food and other essential resources are invalid. Our youth are our future and our legacy so Paladin Movies International produced an edutainment documentary *Please Steal These Ideas,* which proves there are solutions for worldwide youth development, that also support and promote community development!

You will find that the complete *Fountain Of Youth Formula*™ has been provided in the last section. Detailed information is provided on life saving cures for HIV/AIDS, Diabetes, and Cancer, and also on how to easily purify the tap water in your home. Tap water is known to be toxic because it is contaminated with poisonous hard metals, and chemicals such as chlorine and chloramine in the USA, Europe, and even in many developing South American and African countries, such as South Africa.

II *LIVE PROOF VIDEO DOCUMENTATION*

1. Natural Cancer Cure? (Vitamin B17) Man Cures Himself Then Thrown In Jail

To be honest I don't have a clue if this cancer cure works or not but this video still makes me very angry. Do used car sales people who sell customers bad cars get locked up and thrown in jail? Has this guy been found guilty of selling his customers bad products and not offering a refund? If not what right does the FDA have to put someone out of business, and in the process deny people who are sick and/or dying the right to try every remedy possible to save their lives?

This guy was thrown in jail 6 or 7 years ago so this is an ongoing problem. Most likely if I were still living in the USA I would not have wrote this *Fountain Of Youth Formula™: Overview Report.* As you will see in the following videos something is rotten in Denmark. Oh sorry... I meant in the USA.

https://www.youtube.com/watch?v=WvKQrATZ6bU

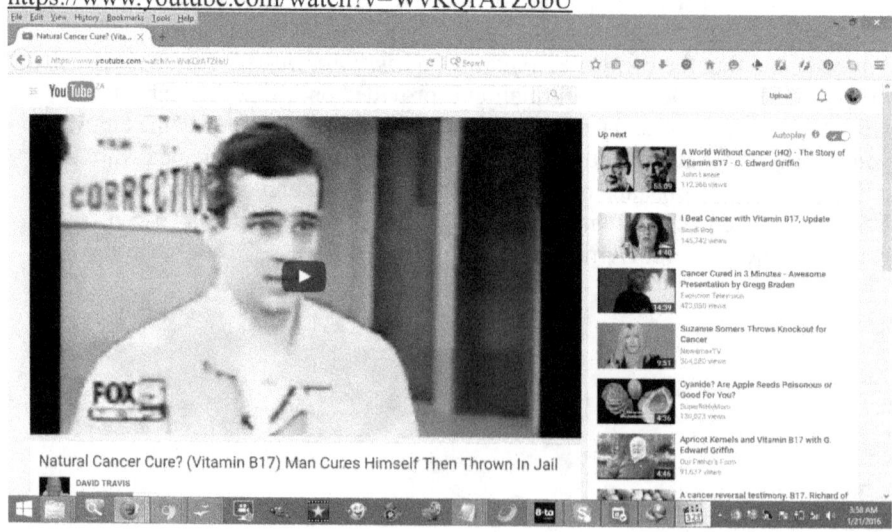

2. Race For The Cure

So far I love this guy Chris although I don't know him and I have never met him! In this video he has the courage to stand up and speak the truth. Chris exposes the Pink Ribbon campaign as a fraudulent business scam so he has probably saved many lives. He's right the Susan G. Komen for the Cure is a waste of your money.

The Susan G. Komen for the Cure program is a multi-million-dollar company with assets totaling over $390 million dollars. Only 20.9% of these funds were reportedly used in the 2009-2010 fiscal year for research, "for the cure", instead of doing research to determine which cure works best. FYI most of the money is spent on "Public Health Education" to encourage screenings for early detection of breast cancer and how Komen gets rich for spreading that message.

https://www.youtube.com/watch?v=jsRVBH3MCQU

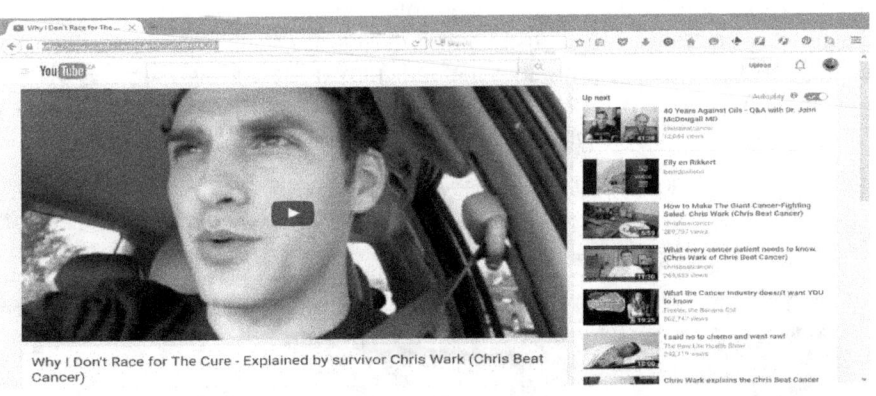

Why I Don't Race for The Cure - Explained by survivor Chris Wark (Chris Beat Cancer)

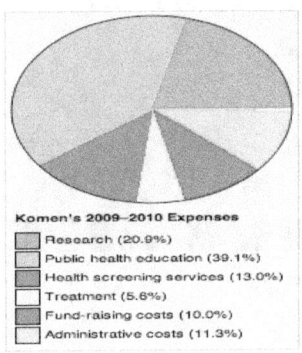

Komen's 2009–2010 Expenses
- Research (20.9%)
- Public health education (39.1%)
- Health screening services (13.0%)
- Treatment (5.6%)
- Fund-raising costs (10.0%)
- Administrative costs (11.3%)

3. Many USA Doctors Should Be In Jail For Murder and/or Insurance Fraud

You may not have heard that the National Cancer Institute admitted millions of patients have been affected by the cancer industry scam: $100 billion a year is spent on toxic chemotherapy for many FAKE diagnoses.

The FDA is locking people up for selling natural cures that the FDA claims are snake oil scams, but have you heard anything about the FDA locking up the scam artists with surgical knives? In the USA people are spending $100 billion per year on toxic chemotherapy treatments and also surgery that mutilates them for no reason, and sadly chemotherapy also causes "chemo brain" side effects.

The National Cancer Institute has publicly admitted that tens of millions of "cancer cases" aren't cancer at all. So tens of millions of people have been diagnosed with "cancer" by crooked oncologists -- and scared into medically unjustified but extremely profitable chemotherapy treatments and surgery. BUT has the FDA locked any doctors or anyone else up? Is the cancer scam in the USA a government sanctioned conspiracy?

(FYI this url is: https://www.youtube.com/watch?v=RJVUuh--_xw)
https://www.youtube.com/watch?v=RJVUuh--_xw

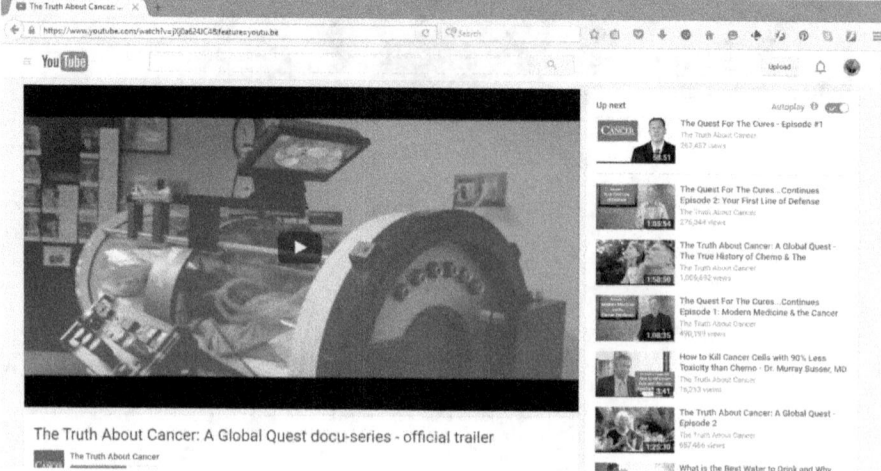

4. I CREATED AIDS to DELIBERATELY DEPOPULATE HUMANITY - Dr Robert Gallo

The London Times ran a front page story, "SMALLPOX VACCINE TRIGGERED AIDS VIRUS," (5/11/87) in which two World Health Organization officials connected the outbreak of AIDS in Africa to the 1977 smallpox vaccination program. This important story never appeared in any mainstream U.S. news media. Nor has the 1979 New York City hepatitis B vaccine trial blood samples containing the first confirmed cases of AIDS.

Dr. Theodore Strecker's research of the literature indicates that the *National Cancer Institute* in collaboration with the *World Health Organization* made the AIDS virus in their laboratories at Fort Detrick in Maryland, USA (now closed). They combined the deadly retroviruses, bovine leukemia virus and sheep *visna virus*, and injected them into human tissue cultures. The result was the AIDS virus.

https://www.youtube.com/watch?v=HgiMqgjS-zM

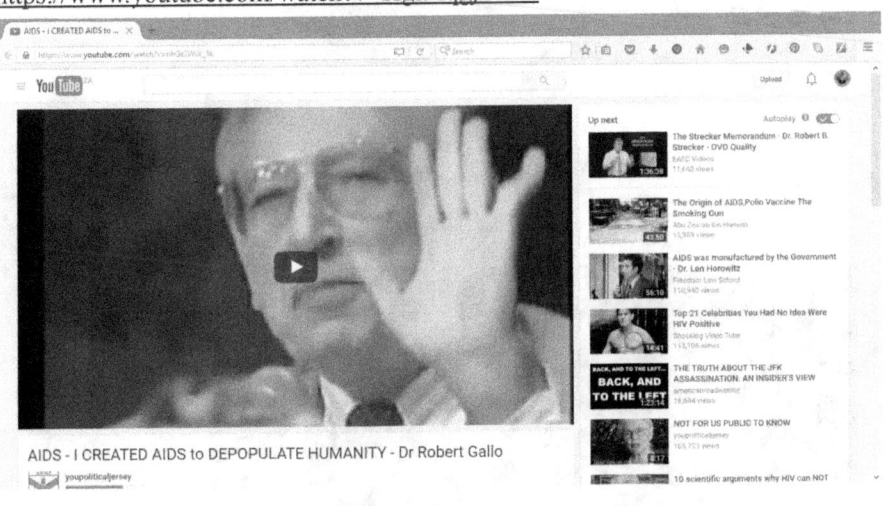

AIDS - I CREATED AIDS to DEPOPULATE HUMANITY - Dr Robert Gallo

youpoliticaljersey

5. The AIDS Scam Parts 1 & 2

More than 200 leading scientists all over the world have spoken up and the evidence is now clear without a doubt the War On AIDS is a profit making scam. AND government agencies in the USA are suppressing information about safe and proven natural cures.

https://www.youtube.com/watch?v=ozU75wgm2O8

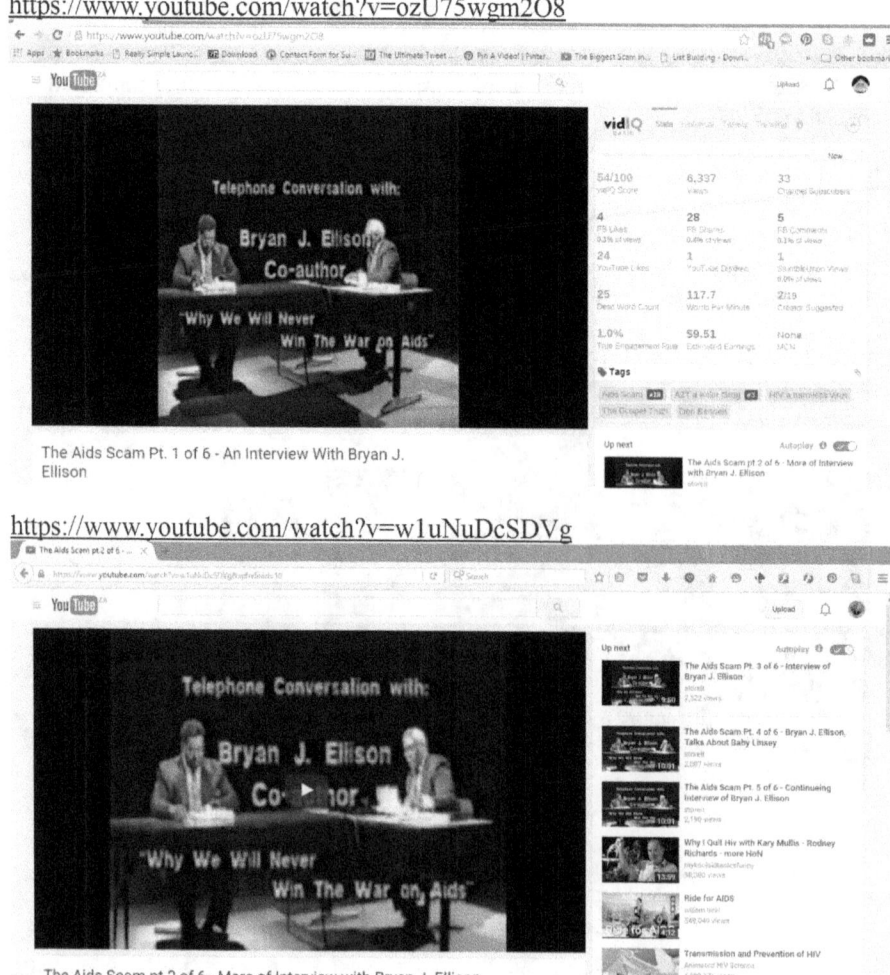

https://www.youtube.com/watch?v=w1uNuDcSDVg

6. Dr. Julian Simon on Resources, Growth and Human Progress

Dr. Julian Simon will forever be a genuine hero for humanity. Dr. Simon had the courage and perseverance to challenge and debunk deceptions by the doomsayers and self-styled environmentalists. While pessimism-pushers such as Lester Brown, Paul Ehrlich, and Al Gore received the mainstream media's reverence Dr. Simon proved so-called theories about resource scarcity due to over population are a myth, and that population growth is a resource.

In his book *The Ultimate Resource 2* Dr. Simon proved that the quantity of resources available at any given time is determined by how creative and energetic people are in extracting resources from the earth, as well as by how creative and energetic we are in devising ways of getting more and more output from each unit of resource. He is a champion for people globally, especially in the developing world, such as in poor countries in Africa that are forced to administer birth control programs designed to depopulate humanity, in order to get grant funding.

https://www.youtube.com/watch?v=mV_38mQ1iG4&list=PL-Jj28S124EOrPLg2aagwfcDJ-8vkY-Sq

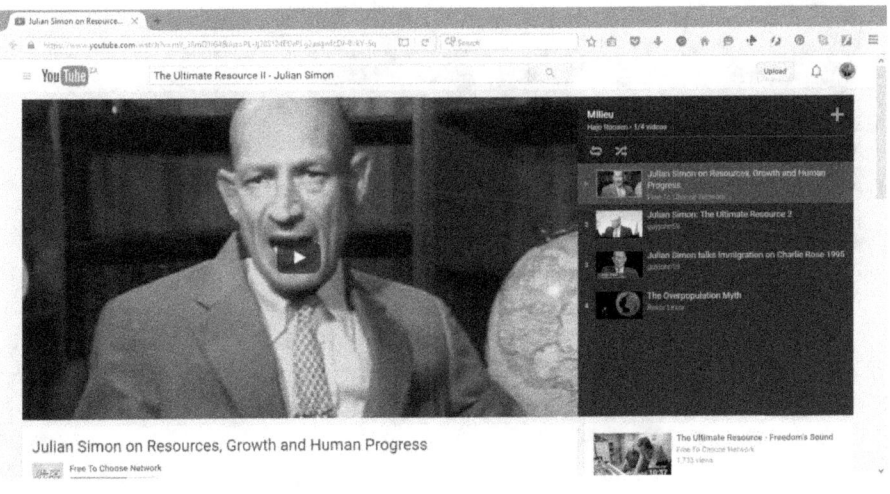

7. Please Steal These Ideas

In addition to diverse video productions Paladin Movies International has developed viable youth programming for youth with skills and talent, that have proven the development of youth and talent also serves to develop the community.

As a result, in 2016 Paladin Movies International is raising funds to launch projects in a rural rea of Durban, South Africa, and in Chicago, Illinois, USA. The overall objective is to produce an edutainment documentary that will provide a model for world-wide youth and community development based on the following edutainment documentary we produced in early 2015.

Our company Motto is "Honesty, Fairness, Doing The Best Job, To Do Good Works Is The Most Sustainable and Profitable Method Of Doing Business."

https://www.youtube.com/watch?v=6tr4fJ7THv0

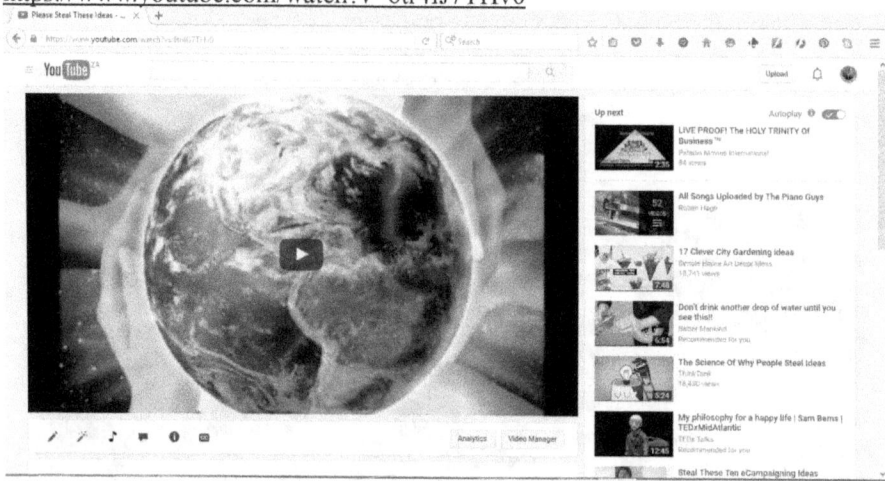

III *Fountain Of Youth Formula*™

You will find that the complete *Fountain Of Youth Formula*™ has been provided in this section of the *Fountain Of Youth Formula*™: *Overview Report*. Below you will also find that very detailed information is provided in this *Fountain Of Youth Formula*™: *Overview Report* on life saving cures for HIV/AIDS and Cancer. The *Fountain Of Youth Formula*™ is based on safe cures that are backed up by scientific principles and proven results. So the good news is there is no scientific basis or requirement in modern society for people to grow old, sickly, and die. The acceptance of the aging process myth in modern society is due to the educational and mass media propaganda and programming, that supports the effort to depopulate humanity.

Fortunately, now it is not only the rich who can afford treatments like the human growth hormone therapy can stay and grow young. Now *YOU* and anyone can stay and/or grow young by using natural and economical products. First you must understand that although human beings have highly developed thinking, superior intelligence and manipulative capabilities our bodies still have physical requirements. Most people seem to believe human beings are different and/or better than common animals that eat, breath, and procreate the same as we do.

In reality we are very much the same and in these modern times I have seen wild monkeys that act more civilized than some people who will do anything and who act like they have rabies, because they are addicted to alcohol, or drugs, or money, and/or racism. Actually the best of us are no different or better than common animals, except that we have hands that have superior manipulation capabilities and brains that have a mostly unused creative power. Possibly most animals might be better than a large percentage of human beings, simply because it is unlikely for any animal without rabies to be sadistic or masochistic.

What distinguishes the best of us from the rest of us is how we use the superior manipulation capabilities of our hands, and also the creative power of our minds and our intelligence for the betterment of our families, friends, society, and the world. Instead of for selfish and exploitative gains. But sadly in modern society upright leadership is lacking. Ronald Reagan was even applauded for saying, "greed is good" when President of the USA. But do not despair, because the solution to the problems we face today have already been provided.

Ideally, even though *The Technological Revolution Is Not Being Televised*™: http://blog.paladinmovies.com/2015/12/newviralsocialtech the Technological Revolution continues to empower people globally. Advances in information technology and digital communication have made information and knowledge accessible to the average person, that has been suppressed and/or only available to wealthy and prominent individuals in the past. You may be surprised to discover that much of the following *Fountain Of Youth Formula*™ has been scientifically tested and proven long ago:

1.) Hair Analysis
Get a Hair Analysis to get a "State Of The Body" report that is more accurate than a blood test to determine nutritional deficiencies and toxins. A blood test may be most useful to determine how to treat the symptoms of illness and to save life in an emergency, but a Hair Analysis is more effective for determining the root cause of illness and disease in order to cure it.

2.) Mega vitamin/mineral therapy
The next most important thing is to use mega vitamin/mineral therapy based the results of your hair analysis, in order to replace the nutrients your body has stopped producing. Although something is better than nothing it is not enough to just buy the best multi vitamin/mineral supplement at the local drug or health food store. Everyone even members of the same family have varying metabolisms, physiology, and body types, that is why a Hair Analysis is required to not only determine your nutritional needs but also identify and rid your body of toxins.

3.) Water Purification
Only the air that we breath is more important for life than water. Water is a living thing that is killed by most modern municipal water purification systems all around the world. Fortunately you can regenerate the water you drink and cook with, first by boiling your water for 20 or 30 minutes to get rid of the chlorine and biological contaminants. Then once your water has cooled it must be filtered through a carbon purification system to get rid of heavy metals and other contaminants.

Next you must add vitamin C to your water to get rid of the chloramine. It is reported that a 1000 mg Vitamin C tablet will neutralize chloramine in an average size bathtub.. But that could vary according to the amount of chloramine that is in your tap water. To be safe I recommend adding 100mg of vitamin C to a gallon of drinking water. Then let your water sit over night to allow it to rejuvenate, drink enough water according to your body weight.

4.) Coconut Oil

2 tablespoons of Coconut Oil per day. Coconut Oil has been reported to be more effective than pharmaceutical drugs in treating *Alzheimer's* Disease. Coconut Oil has been called a super food, because of its superior content of nutrition and medicinal healing capabilities.

5.) Carrot juice

Drink 1 quart of freshly made carrot juice with half a small beet per day. Carrot juice is another super food due to it's high content of nutrition and medicinal healing capabilities.

6.) Nigella sativa seed oil

1 tablespoon or 2 grams of Nigella sativa seed oil daily depending on age, body weight, and medical condition. Scientific research has determined that Nigella sativa seed oil is an effective treatment for the following diseases, but some people believe this list is just the tip of the iceberg. Get specific advise from a certified naturopathic practitioner.

1. Type 2 diabetes

2. Epilepsy

3. Colon Cancer

4. MRSA

5. Protection Against Heart Attack Damage

6. Breast Cancer

7. Brain Cancer

8. Leukemia

9. Brain Damage from Lead

10. Oral Cancer

7.) Selenium

400mg per day of selenium has been proven to be a cure for HIV/AIDS that is similar to the TB cure. Again depending on age, body weight, and medical condition. Get specific advise from a certified naturopathic practitioner.

8.) **Oxygenation Therapy The Cure For Virtually All Diseases**

The information on how to use the Hydrogen Peroxide (HP) oxygenation therapy to cure illness and disease was provided by Madison Cavanaugh's *The One-Minute Cure* book: http://blog.paladinmovies.com/2016/01/oneminutecure HP oxygenation therapy is commonly used to oxygenate the body all around the world, due to the miraculous health benefits except in the USA. One of the best things about the HP oxygenation therapy is that when handled and used properly it can be safely self administered at home for less than 2 cents per day.

An oxygenation therapy that is medically administered called ozone therapy, has been proven to be powerful enough to cure the most deadly diseases, and even AIDS. Most of the benefits of medically administered ozone oxygenation therapy can also be attributed to the self administration of HP oxygenation therapy, because ozone is transformed into hydrogen peroxide in the body.

Deadly diseases caused by hostile micro-organisms are eradicated by hydrogen peroxide the same way they are eliminated with an ozone blood infusion. HP oxygenation therapy is easily administered at home but it also kills viruses and other pathogens throughout the body and it also revitalizes normal cells due to the boost of oxygen.

Unlike prescription medications there are practically no adverse side affects or known risks when using HP oxygenation therapy. BUT again hydrogen peroxide must be handled and used properly, OR it can be deadly and even fatal. As a result before you decide to self-administer HP oxygenation therapy it is critical that you understand that there are many different grades of hydrogen peroxide available on the market, but only one grade is safe for human consumption and it must be handled very carefully.

The only grade of hydrogen peroxide that's suitable for human consumption is the **35% FOOD GRADE**, which must not be confused with the 35% Technical Grade. You can buy **35% FOOD GRADE** hydrogen peroxide that is suitable for human consumption in pints, quarts, gallons, and drums at some mom and pop or alternative drugstores. If none are available where you may live you can use google to find out where you can buy **35% FOOD GRADE** hydrogen peroxide on the Internet.

IMPORTANT NOTICE: The **35% FOOD GRADE** hydrogen peroxide needs to be diluted before being taken internally. Also as mentioned previously **35% FOOD GRADE** hydrogen peroxide must be handled very carefully. It is highly flammable and it will even will burn your skin if you if you come in contact with it. If you spill any on your skin you must immediately wash your skin thoroughly. **Also beware that consuming 35% FOOD GRADE hydrogen peroxide before dilution is fatal, and even consuming 10% strength hydrogen peroxide will cause neurological damage.**

To be extra careful when handling hydrogen peroxide it is recommended that you use rubber gloves. It is also suggested that the best way to dilute hydrogen peroxide properly is to use a glass bottle with an eyedropper cap. Once you fill the glass bottle label it "**35% Food Grade** Hydrogen Peroxide" to prevent accidental undiluted usage.

In addition, the **35% Food Grade** hydrogen peroxide should be stored in a refrigerator out of the reach of children. Madison Cavanaugh provides excellent therapies for the rapid cure of many diseases in her book *The One-Minute Cure.* The basic maintenance dose for the use of the HP oxygenation therapy is to drink 1 drop of **35% FOOD GRADE** hydrogen peroxide, that has been diluted with 6 to 8 ounces of distilled water 3 times per day. **DO NOT USE TAP WATER BECAUSE IT IS WITH CHLORINE & CHLORAMINE.**

Currently the cost for **35% FOOD GRADE** hydrogen peroxide is very inexpensive at approximately $13 for a 16 oz. bottle. So the maintenance therapy of 1 drop in 6 to 8 ounces of distilled water 3 times a day will only cost approximately 1½ cents per day. Of course as this information spreads and becomes common knowledge the price will increase. Just like chicken wings are now the most expensive part of the chicken, but they were the cheapest until they became the most popular part of the chicken.

Anyway if you find the taste of diluted hydrogen peroxide unpleasant you can also dilute **35% FOOD GRADE** hydrogen peroxide with six to eight ounces of milk, aloe vera, or watermelon juice instead of water. In addition to diluting hydrogen peroxide with chlorine and chloramine free (preferably distilled) water, it is important that you take the HP oxygenation therapy on an empty stomach. The best time is 1 hour before eating or 3 hours after eating.

FYI water that has been purified with chlorine and chloramine is reported to aggravate and/or cause of many illnesses including the following conditions:

A.) Increase in the incidence of allergies and asthma
cause bladder and rectal cancer
B.) Damage to airways and soft tissues
C.) Skin and eye irritation
D.) Reduced beneficial gut flora
E.) High concentrations also cause fluid in the lungs

Especially if you are currently sick and even if you are not it is advised to start using the HP oxygenation therapy with the advice and guidance or a certified natural health practitioner. As long as you are healthy if you become nauseated you can reduce the therapy to once or twice per day until your body adjusts, then increase to the recommended 3 times per day. FYI it is not uncommon to experience nausea, fatigue, diarrhea, cold or flu-like symptoms, or skin eruptions as your body expels large amounts of toxins and dead cells.

Your body may go through what is commonly called a "healing crisis" as your body reacts to the removal of disease-causing or toxic conditions. So don't be alarmed and stop the therapy if you feel uncomfortable for a few days, that means the HP oxygenation therapy is working. Remember that your body is getting rid of disease and toxins that were acquired over many years.

In her book *The One-Minute Cure* Madison Cavanaugh also describes how HP oxygenation therapy has been successfully used in the treatment of emphysema, which is commonly considered to be incurable and terminal. In addition, Madison may share as many as a dozen other different ways HP oxygenation therapy can be used to cure a seemingly unlimited number of other diseases and ailments.

She correctly points out that most people are only familiar with hydrogen peroxide bought over-the-counter at the local drug store. So fortunately for us Madison has written *The One-Minute Cure* because as she rightly shares, "Not everyone is aware that it (hydrogen peroxide) is also a naturally occurring substance (in the body)."

"A mother's breast milk, for instance, contains high amounts of hydrogen peroxide, and the first milk (colostrum) contains even higher amounts. This has been shown as one of the main reasons why breast milk stimulates an infant's immune system and activates metabolic processes."

"Throughout the (our lives) life cycle, the human body produces hydrogen peroxide constantly. The immune system uses this naturally occurring hydrogen peroxide to oxidize foreign invaders (phagocytosis)—parasites, viruses, bacteria, yeast and fungus, thereby warding off disease. However, oxygen deficient bodies are unable to produce enough hydrogen peroxide on their own. That is why oxygen therapy, especially through hydrogen peroxide (HP oxygenation therapy) administration, is extremely important."

9.) *Growing Young & Regaining Youth*

Research has proven that the daily regime above can cure most all diseases. In order to regain youth and grow young again the next steps are required. Regular workouts 3 to 5 days per week that induce intense sweating for at least 20 minutes non stop. Swimming and/or rebounding (jumping on a trampoline) are both excellent exercises to condition your body to start a regular vigorous work out program. It will take time to build up the stamina for intense work outs and it is also recommended to consult a physician before beginning a work out program.

To grow young again it is also most important to stop eating red meat and especially pork. If you are serious about growing young you must understand that dead foods can not make you grow young again. So in order to grow young most rapidly it is best to become a vegan or a vegetarian, or at least to only consume fish and fowl.

CONCLUSION

Your health is your most important asset so firstly the *Fountain Of Youth Formula*™: *Overview Report* has focused on providing the best information available for you to cure yourself by natural means. Of course it is expected that once you become healthier, and you are on the path to regain your youth most likely you will also want to buy the *Fountain Of Youth Formula*™ eBook, that will be published on or before Valentine's Day 2016!

Readers who appreciate the *Fountain Of Youth Formula*™: *Overview Report* and have found it to be useful and helpful for naturally regaining their health and youth will be glad to know the The *Fountain Of Youth Formula*™ eBook will provide much more indepth and comprehensive coverage on how you can actually grow young by using the *Fountain Of Youth Formula*™. Here are some of resources that you will find in the *Fountain Of Youth Formula*™ eBook:

- Full details on a scientific work out method, that has been called the most effective system for rapid body building and body sculpturing.

- Free download link for the Coconut Oil Cures eBook: The Best Kept Secret for Anti-Aging, Weight Loss, Disease Prevention and Health Restoration.

- DIY plan for making your own water purification filtration system, for clean water that's healthier than most bottled water and cheaper than buying filters.

- Special formulas to super charge the natural ingredients that are recommended and used in *Fountain Of Youth Formula*™.

- A Mega vitamin/mineral therapy guide.

- A FREE copy of *The Science Of Getting Rich* book by Wallace D. Wattles, Wattles book provides tested and proven wisdom on how to be rich in health, intelligence, and spirituality in a way that automatically attracts money to yourself.

- A FREE Guide On 6 Proven Health Benefits for Using Apple Cider Vinegar

You will probably be glad to know that you can also get a 50% Off Coupon to buy the *The Fountain Of Youth Formula*™ eBook for Half Price! After you have read *The Fountain Of Youth Formula*™: *Overview Report* just go back and post a short honest testimonial review in the comments section of the HotZone Video Blog at: http://blog.paladinmovies.com/overviewreport We will send your coupon code to the email address you provided.

The Half Price Special Is A Limited Time Special Offer That Will End Before *The Fountain Of Youth Formula*™ eBook Is Published On Valentines Day February 14, 2016. So don't wait – Hurry Back! Be Healthy, Live Long, Do Good Works & Prosper!

Best Regards, Ron Benson

For Hot Updates Follow @GorillaShooting
https://twitter.com/GorillaShooting

SCIENTIFIC RESEARCH

"10 Facts about Diabetes" World Health Organization
http://who.int/features/factfiles/diabetes/facts/en/index1.html

"America's Health Rankings"
http://www.americashealthrankings.org/all/diabetes#sthash.hb3kznVW.dpuf

"Benefits of Coconut Oil for Thyroid"
http://www.coconutoilfacts.org/coconut-oil-thyroid.php

"Coconut and health—a literature review"
Secretariat of the Pacific Community 2003. http://www.spc.int/lifestyle/

"Type 1 diabetes in urban children skyrockets, increasing by 70% in
children under age 5" Science Daily, January 22, 2013
http://www.sciencedaily.com/releases/2013/01/130122111512.htm

"U.S. study looks into the benefits of coconut oil on patients with Alzheimer's"
CTV News. http://www.ctvnews.ca/health/health-headlines/u-s-study-looks-into-
thebenefits-of-coconut-oil-on-patients-with-alzheimer-s-1.1491406

Calbom, C., and Shilhavy, B. "How to Help Your Thyroid with Virgin Coconut
Oil" http://articles.mercola.com/sites/articles/archive/2003/11/08/thyroid-
healthpart-two.aspx

Centers for Disease Control. "Facts about Obesity in the United States"
http://www.cdc.gov/pdf/facts_about_obesity_in_the_united_states.pdf

Gupta, Dr. Sanjay. "If we are what we eat, Americans are corn and soy"
http://www.cnn.com/2007/HEALTH/diet.fitness/09/22/kd.gupta.column/index.htm
l

McNiff, Tom. "One wife's crusade: Coconut oil helped husband with Alzheimer's"
The Gainesville Sun, March, 2013
Meletis, Chris D. "Alzheimer's: Type 3 Diabetes?"
http://www.wholehealthinsider.com/newsletter/alzheimers-type-3-diabetes/

Newport, Dr. Mary. "What If There Was a Cure for Alzheimer's Disease and No One Knew?"
http://www.coconutketones.com/whatifcure.pdf

Walling, Elizabeth. "Coconut Oil Can Promote Weight Loss by Increasing Metabolism Naturally"
http://www.naturalnews.com/026808_oil_coconut.html

"Hydrogen Peroxide Kills Staphylococcus Aureus By Reacting With Staphylococcal Iron To Form Hydroxyl Radical"
John E. Repine, Richard B. Fox and Elaine M. Berger
The Journal of Biological Chemistry
July 25, 1981
Volume 256 Number 14
Pages 7094-7096

"Survival of Nosocomial Bacterial and Spores on Surfaces and Inactivation by Hydrogen Peroxide Vapor"
Jonathan A. Otter and Gary L. French
Journal of Clinical Microbiology
January, 2009
Volume 47
Number 1
Pages 205-207

"Inactivation of Animal and Human Prions by Hydrogen Peroxide Gas Plasma Sterilization"
Rogez-Kreuz C, Yousfi R, Soufflet C, Quadrio I, Yan ZX, Huyot V, Aubenque C, Destrez P, Roth K, Roberts C, Favero M, Clayette P.
Infect. Control Hosp. Epidemiol.
August, 2009
Volume 30 (8)
Pages 769-777

CANCER
"A Method of Destroying a Malignant Rat Tumour In Vivo"
R.A. Holman
Nature
May 18, 1957

Number 4568
Page 1033

"Application of Hydrogen Peroxide Infusion to Maxillary Cancer"
Hiroshi Sasaki, Tadao Wakutani, Sikayuki Oda and Yasuo Yamasaki
Yonago Acta Medica
October, 1967
Volume 11, Number 3
Pages 141-149

Journal of Experimental Medicine
July, 1980
Volume 152
Pages 198-2082

www.ingramcontent.com/pod-product-compliance
Lightning Source LLC
Chambersburg PA
CBHW070303190526
45169CB00004B/1509